THE
Skinny SLOW
COOKER
VEGETARIAN
RECIPE BOOK

MEAT FREE RECIPES UNDER 200, 300 AND 400 CALORIES

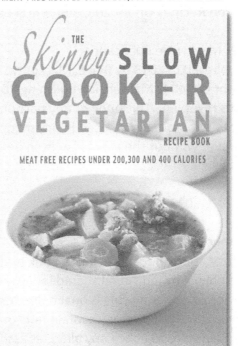

THE
Skinny SLOW
COOKER
VEGETARIAN
RECIPE BOOK

MEAT FREE RECIPES UNDER 200, 300 AND 400 CALORIES

The Skinny Slow Cooker Vegetarian Recipe Book
Meat Free Recipes Under 200, 300 & 400 Calories

A Bell & Mackenzie Publication
First published in 2013 by Bell & Mackenzie Publishing
Copyright © Bell & Mackenzie Publishing 2013

ISBN 978-1-909855-00-7

Disclaimer
The information and advice in this book is intended as
a guide only. Any individual should independently seek
the advice of a health professional before embarking
on a diet. Some recipes may contain nuts or traces of
nuts. Those suffering from any allergies associated with
nuts should avoid any recipes containing nuts or nut
based oils.

Contents

Introduction   8
Preparation   8
Nutrition   9
Low Cost   9
Using Your Slow Cooker: A Few Things   9
Meals   **11**
Wild Mushroom Stroganoff   12
Nightshade Thai Curry   14
Creamy Korma   15
Veggie Chickpea Curry   16
Slow Spanish Tombet   17
Caribbean Spiced Sweet Potatoes   18
Shepherd-less Lentil Pie   19
Sloppy Joes   20
Chickpea Cattia   21
Baked Potatoes & Butternut Squash   22
Lean Green Risotto   23
Hand To Mouth Tex Mex Tacos   24
Luxury Macaroni Cheese   25
Pomodoro Pasta Sauce   26
Risi e Bisi   27
Bean, Potato & Cheese Stew   28
Apple Root Stew   29
Berber Rice Baked Peppers   30
Double Potato Casserole   31
Beetroot Bean Salad Topping   32
Spiced Sweet Potatoes & Eggs   33
Kale & Lentil Supper   34
Creamed Cheese & Sweetcorn Supper   35
Capsicum Mexican Chilli   37
Lemon & Hazelnut Brocoli   38
Garlic & Broccoli Breadcrumb Pasta   39

Contents

Sweet Beans & Spinach 40
Vegetarian Sausage & Spinach With Gnocchi 41
Basil, Peppers & Gnocchi 42
Mushroom Ragu 43
Basil Zucchini Bake 44
Paprika Potatoes 45
Tomato & Garlic Mushrooms 46
Fennel Risotto 47
Boston Bean Dream 48
Lentil Dhal 50
Butter Beans & Almond Stew 51
Soups **53**
Corn & Potato Chowder 54
Barley & Chestnut Mushroom Soup 55
St. Patrick's Day Soup 56
Asian Hot Soup 57
Zucchini Soup 58
Squash, Basil & Tomato Soup 59
Spicy Carrot Soup 60
Flagelot & Savoy Soup 61
Parsnip & Coconut Milk Soup 62
Spinach & Haricot Soup 63
Appetisers/Snacks **65**
Sweet & Salty Almond Snack or Killer Salad! 66
Bean, Rosemary & Roasted Garlic Dip 68
Italian Mushrooms 69
Hummus bi Tahini 71
Braised Garlic Sauerkraut 72
Slow Cooked Corn 73
Spicy Creamed Spinach 74
Apple Sauce 75
Nacho, Bean & Onion Dip 76

Contents

Spiced Red Cabbage & Apple 77

Succotash 78

Parmesan Style Green Beans 79

Sweet & Sour Savoy 80

Silky Leeks & Peas 81

Creamy Celery & Walnuts 82

Marmalade Carrots 83

Honey Roasted Vegetables 84

Desserts **85**

Warming Spiced Apples 86

Cinnamon Apples 87

Buckle Berry Cobbler 88

Bread Pudding 89

Rice Pudding 91

Citrus Slice 92

Stewed Rhubarb & Cream 93

Rum Bananas 94

Apricots & Pistachios 95

Ginger Plums With Greek Yoghurt 96

Breakfasts **97**

Spanish Tortilla 98

Multi Grain Breakfast 99

Fruit Granola 100

Morning Risotto 101

Vanilla Prunes 102

Banana Porridge Oats 103

A Real Cooked Breakfast 104

Conversion Chart 106

Review & Other CookNation Books **108**

THE *Skinny* SLOW COOKER VEGETARIAN
RECIPE BOOK

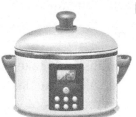

INTRODUCTION

Introduction

Welcome to The Skinny Slow Cooker Vegetarian Recipe Book: 40 Meat Free Recipes Under 200, 300 And 400 Calories from the Kitchen Collection on Kindle.

Whether you are a vegetarian or just love vegetables, this collection of easy to prepare and delicious low-calorie vegetarian recipes will 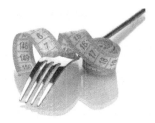 help you make inexpensive, healthy, meat free meals with the minimum of fuss.

The recipes are simple and easy to follow with inexpensive fresh and seasonal ingredients and are packed full of flavour and goodness so you can enjoy maximum taste with minimum calories.

Preparation

None of these recipes should take more than 10-15 minutes to prepare. All vegetables should be cut into even sized pieces. Although root vegetables can take longer to cook, generally make sure everything is bite-sized and washed before use. Remember that unlike meat, vegetables do not produce their own juices to cook in so it is important to add the required liquid/ stock to each recipe (we've covered this in each list of ingredients). Also, slow cooking with veg means you can happily use canned and frozen vegetables too. Just remember that frozen veg will reduce the temperature of the slow cooker and therefore you will need to increase overall cooking time if substituting frozen for fresh. Where our recipes use beans we have used canned beans for ease. Dried beans are fine too but will require overnight soaking.

Nutrition

All of the recipes in this collection are balanced low calorie family meals under 400 calories which should keep you feeling full and help you avoid snacking inbetween 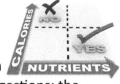 meals. All recipes have serving suggestions; the calories noted are per serving of the recipe ingredients only so bear that in mind.

Low Cost

Slow cooking is a wonderful way to produce delicious meals without spending a fortune, plus the slow cooker process retains the goodness and nutrition of the vegetables so both your purse and your waistline benefit. We've made sure not to include lots of one-off ingredients which are only for a single recipe and never used again. All the herbs and spices listed can be used in multiple recipes throughout the book.

Using Your Slow Cooker: A Few Things

All cooking times are a guide. Make sure you get to know your own slow cooker so that you can adjust timings accordingly to ensure your meals are properly cooked through.

A spray of one-cal cooking oil in the cooker before adding ingredients will help with cleaning or you can buy liners.

Be confident with your cooking. Feel free to use substitutes to suit your own taste and don't let a missing herb or spice stop you making a meal - you'll almost always be able to find something to replace it.

THE Skinny SLOW COOKER VEGETARIAN

RECIPE BOOK

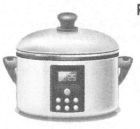

MEALS

Wild Mushroom Stroganoff

Serves 4

101
CALORIES
PER SERVING

Ingredients:

675g/1 ½lb wild mixed mushrooms, sliced
2 large onions, chopped
4 garlic cloves, crushed
2 tsp smoked paprika
250ml/1 cup vegetable stock/broth

1 400g/14oz tin low fat condensed mushroom soup
Knob butter
3 tbsp freshly chopped flat leaf parsley
Salt & pepper to taste

Method:

Add all the ingredients to the slow cooker, except the parsley. Season well, cover and leave to cook on high for 2-3 hours or low 4-5 hours. Ensure the mushrooms are tender. Sprinkle with chopped parsley and serve with pasta or rice and a spoon of low fat natural yoghurt.

The more exciting the mushrooms, the better this dish is going to taste. Use whatever is available; a combination of portobella, shitake, morel, oyster and enoki would be fantastic but don't be put off if you can only get regular varieties.

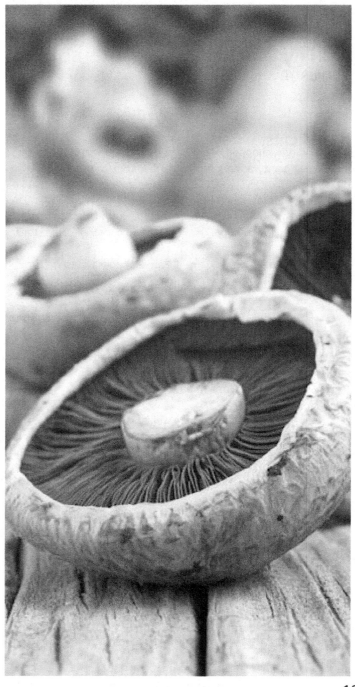

Nightshade Thai Curry

Serves 4

Ingredients:

3 large onions, chopped
1 large egg plant / aubergine, diced
200g/7oz potatoes, diced
425g/15oz mushrooms, sliced
1 green chilli, finely chopped
3 cloves garlic, crushed
1 tsp ground ginger

3 tbsp green thai curry paste
1 tbsp tomato puree
2 tbsp groundnut or vegetable oil
1 tbsp plain/all purpose flour
750ml/3 cups vegetable stock/ broth
Salt & pepper to taste

Method:

Gently saute the onions, aubergine, potatoes and mushrooms in the oil for a couple of minutes. Add all the other ingredients (except stock) and stir for a minute or two longer.

Add the vegetable stock, combine well and bring to a high heat before transferring to the slow cooker. Cover and leave to cook on a low heat for 4-5 hours or 2-3 hours on high; or until the potatoes are tender. Add a little more stock during cooking if needed, or if it needs thickening remove the lid and leave to cook on high for a further 45 minutes or until you get the desired consistency.

Serve with chopped onion salad, brown rice or naan bread.

Nightshade is just one of the many local names for aubergine/egg plant. Loved by vegetarians for its ability to absorb large amounts of cooking sauces, the nightshade is twinned here with potatoes to give a lovely, full and rich dish.

Creamy Korma
Serves 4

Ingredients:

1 tbsp vegetable oil
2 large onions, chopped
3 cardamom pods
2 tsp ground cumin
2 tsp ground coriander
1 tsp ground ginger
½ tsp turmeric
1 green chili, chopped (add more if you prefer)
2 garlic cloves, crushed

225g/8oz carrots, sliced
225g/8oz cauliflower florets
225g/8oz courgettes/zucchini, sliced
225g/8oz potatoes, cubed
225g/8oz frozen peas
500ml/2 cups vegetable stock/broth
250ml/1 cup fat free Greek yoghurt

Method:

Give the cardamom pods a bash, then add the onion, garlic, oil and all the dry spices to a frying pan and leave to cook gently for a few minutes. Add the chilli and vegetables (except the peas) and leave to cook for another minute or two then remove to the slow cooker. Leave to cook on a low heat for 3-4 hours with the lid tightly shut or 2-3 hours on high. 30 minutes before the end add the peas. Add a little more stock during cooking if needed, or if it needs thickening remove the lid and leave to cook on high for a further 45 minutes or until you get the desired consistency. Ensure the vegetables are tender, stir in the yoghurt and serve.

Lovely with rice, ground almonds and chopped coriander/cilantro.

A characteristic Indian dish, korma's roots can be traced back to the 16th century. Defined as a dish where meat or vegetables are braised with water/stock and yoghurt. This vegetarian version is perfect when you fancy a tasty curry without too much 'kick'.

15

Veggie Chickpea Curry
Serves 4

234 CALORIES PER SERVING

Ingredients:

2 400g/14oz tins chickpeas, drained
2 onions, chopped
3 tbsp tomato puree/paste
2 cloves garlic, crushed
1 tsp fresh grated ginger (or use ½ teaspoon of ginger powder)
1 tbsp garam masala
1 tsp each of ground cumin & coriander/cilantro
2 tsp turmeric
½ tsp chilli powder
75g/3oz fresh spinach
2 tbsp lemon juice
500ml/2 cups vegetable stock/broth
Pinch salt

Method:

Combine all the ingredients, except the lemon juice and spinach, in the slow cooker. Cover and leave to cook on low for 4-6 hours or on high for 2-4 hours. Ensure the chickpeas are cooked though. Add a little more stock during cooking if needed, or if it needs thickening remove the lid and leave to cook on high for a further 45 minutes or until you get the desired consistency. Stir in the lemon juice and spinach; serve with rice and naan bread.

Chickpeas have been used in cooking for many hundreds of years. If you prefer your spinach well-cooked add earlier in the recipe. The method here will leave it with a bit of crunchy freshness.

Slow Spanish Tombet

Serves 4

Ingredients:

2 fresh aubergines/eggplant, cubed

2 courgettes , cut into strips

200g/7oz fresh tomatoes, cubed

2 (bell) peppers, sliced

5 tbsp tomato puree/paste

2 large red onions, 1 chopped, 1 sliced

1 tsp each of dried marjoram, basil & thyme

1 tsp paprika

1 tsp capers, chopped

Handful pitted black olives, chopped

3 garlic cloves, crushed

250ml/1 cup vegetable stock/broth

1 tsp salt

1 tsp sugar

1 tbsp olive oil

3 tbsp freshly chopped basil

Method:

Combine all ingredients, except the fresh basil, in the slow cooker, cover and leave to cook on low for 4-5 hours or high for 2-3 hours. Add a little more stock during cooking if needed, or if it needs thickening remove the lid and leave to cook on high for a further 45 minutes or until you get the desired consistency.

Tombet is the Spanish version of the French classic ratatouille. This is lovely served with Spanish toast; which is simply rough cut farmhouse bread toasted and rubbed with garlic, salt & olive oil.

Caribbean Spiced Sweet Potatoes

Serves 4

225 CALORIES PER SERVING

Ingredients:

400g/14oz sweet potatoes, cubed
1 onion, chopped
125g/4oz green beans, sliced
1 200g/7oz tin black beans
½ cup /120ml vegetable stock/ broth
½ cup/120ml coconut milk

2 garlic cloves, crushed
½ tsp each cayenne pepper, nutmeg, cinnamon
1 tsp each dried onion powder, thyme, parsley, paprika & brown sugar
Salt & pepper to taste

Method:

Combine all ingredients in the slow cooker. Cover and leave to cook on low for 4-6 hours or until the sweet potatoes are tender. Add a little more stock during cooking if needed, or if it needs thickening remove the lid and leave to cook on high for a further 45 minutes or until you get the desired consistency.

For an authentic taste of the Caribbean serve with fried plantain and chunky coleslaw.

Shepherd-less Lentil Pie

Serves 4

250 CALORIES PER SERVING

Ingredients:

1 tbsp olive oil
1 onions, chopped
2 carrots, diced
2 stalks celery, chopped
1 garlic clove, crushed
75g/3oz mushrooms , sliced
1 bay leaf
1 tbsp dried thyme
100g/3 ½ oz dried green lentils
(soaked overnight)

60ml/ ¼ cup red wine
2 tbsp vegetarian
worcestershire sauce
250ml/1 cup vegetable stock/
broth
3 tbsp tomato purée
1 ½ lb / 680g mashed potato to
top the pie

Method:

Gently sauté the onions, celery, carrots, garlic and herbs in the oil for a few minutes. Remove to the slow cooker and combine well with all the other ingredients, except the mashed potato. Season, cover and leave to cook on low for 4-5 hours or high for 2-3 hours. Add a little more stock during cooking if needed, or if it needs thickening remove the lid and leave to cook on high for a further 45 minutes or until you get the desired consistency. Remove from the slow cooker and place in an ovenproof dish. Top with the mashed potato and brown under the grill for a few minutes.

Lovely served with peas and spring greens dressed with garlic oil.

Sloppy Joes
Serves 4

Ingredients:

200g/7oz lentils (soaked overnight)
1 400g/14oz tin chopped tomatoes
1 tsp olive oil
1 onion, chopped
1 green pepper, chopped
1 tsp chilli powder
½ tsp garlic powder

½ tsp mustard powder
250ml/1 cup vegetable stock/broth
2 tbsp soy sauce
125g/4oz soy meat (TVP / Quorn mince)
3 tbsp ketchup or BBQ sauce
Salt & pepper to taste

Method:

Gently sauté the onions & pepper in a frying pan with the oil for a few minutes then combine all the ingredients into the slow cooker, cover and cook on low for 6-8 hours or until the lentils are tender. Add a little more stock during cooking if needed, or if it needs thickening remove the lid and leave to cook on high for a further 45 minutes or until you get the desired consistency.
Serve with toasted sandwich buns, lettuce & onion.

An American classic, 'Sloppy Joes' can still be enjoyed by the meat-free amongst us. This recipe uses soy meat but that could be substituted for a basic bean mix; soak overnight whatever store cupboard beans you have and fry them with some garlic, onion and a little flaxseed.

Chickpea Cattia
Serves 4

240
CALORIES
PER SERVING

Ingredients:

1 tsp each of ground cumin, turmeric, garam masala & paprika

½ tsp each of sea salt, ground coriander/cilantro, ginger & black pepper

2 tbsp ground nut or vegetable oil

1 large onion, chopped

250ml/1 cup vegetable stock/broth

2 fresh tomatoes, chopped

2 cloves garlic, crushed

2 400g/14oz tins chickpeas, drained

Handful pitted black olives

200g/7oz butternut squash or pumpkin, cubed

1 bay leaf

2 tbsp lemon juice

75g/3oz vegetarian feta style cheese, crumbled

Method:

Combine all the ingredients into the slow cooker, except the feta cheese and lemon juice. Cover, season and leave to cook on low for 5-6 hours or high for 3-4 hours or until the vegetables are tender. Add a little more stock during cooking if needed, or if it needs thickening remove the lid and leave to cook on high for a further 45 minutes or until you get the desired consistency. After cooking stir in the lemon juice and feta cheese and serve with a dollop of low fat yoghurt and rice if you like.

Cattia is the ancient Latin word from which casserole has its origins. This chickpea version is jam packed with spices along with some lemon zest to lift the dish.

Baked Potatoes & Butternut Squash
Serves 4

260 CALORIES PER SERVING

Ingredients:

600g/1lb 5oz baking potatoes
2 whole butternut squash
1 tbsp olive oil
1 tsp rock salt

2 tsp slow fat 'butter' spread
½ tsp each ground nutmeg &
cinnamon

Method:

Stab the potatoes with a fork and rub with olive oil and rock salt.
Wrap each in foil and place into the slow cooker along with the
whole butternut squashes. Cover tightly and leave to cook on high
for 3-5 hours or low for 6-8 hours; or until both the potatoes and
squash are tender.
Remove from the slow cooker. Cut open the squashes and scoop
out seeds. Remove the flesh and mix with the butter, nutmeg and
cinnamon to make a creamy pulp. Cut open the potatoes and
serve with the squash pulp and a green salad.

*Although they are delicious there's nothing new
about cooking baked potatoes in the slow cooker, but
twinning them with sweet baked butternut squash
adds a new twist.*

Lean Green Risotto
Serves 4

Ingredients:

1 tbsp olive oil
1 tsp low fat 'butter' spread
1 large onion, chopped
2 cloves of garlic, crushed
250g/9oz risotto rice
1lt/4 cups vegetable stock/broth

1 tbsp vegetarian green pesto
75g/3oz green beans, chopped
75g/3oz peas
75g/3oz fresh spinach, chopped

Method:

Saute the onion in the oil and butter for a few minutes. Add the risotto rice to the pan and make sure each grain is coated well with the oil and butter. Transfer to the slow cooker and combine all the ingredients. Cover, season and leave to cook on high for 2-3 hours until tender. The risotto may need a little more stock during cooking, or if it needs thickening remove the lid and leave to cook on high for a further 45 minutes or until you get the desired consistency.

Serve with a basil garnish and plain rocket salad with vegetarian parmesan style cheese shavings.

Usually served as a first course in Italy, this veggie pesto version makes a beautiful main course.

Hand To Mouth Tex Mex Tacos
Serves 4

Ingredients:

1 400g/14oz tin black beans, drained
1 400g/14oz tin chopped tomatoes
75g/3oz frozen sweetcorn
1 courgette/zucchini chopped
1 green (bell) pepper, finely chopped
1 tsp paprika

½ tsp each chilli powder & garlic powder
1 tsp each oregano, thyme, cumin and onion powder
125g/4oz rice
250ml/1 cup vegetable stock/broth
Salt & pepper to taste

Method:

Combine all the ingredients into the slow cooker. Season, cover and leave to cook on low for 6-8 hours or high 4-6 hours; or until the rice is tender. Add a little more stock during cooking if needed, or if it needs thickening remove the lid and leave to cook on high for a further 45 minutes or until you get the desired consistency.

Serve with your choice of taco shells, avocado, lettuce, salsa, cheese, onions or sour cream.

Tacos are traditionally eaten with hands not utensils and this gorgeous mix should be no different. Enjoy with friends who don't mind messy eaters!

Luxury Macaroni Cheese
Serves 4

380 CALORIES PER SERVING

Ingredients:

300g/11oz macaroni pasta
200g/7oz grated vegetarian reduced fat cheddar cheese
2 tsp dijon mustard
120ml/ ½ cup evaporated milk
385ml/1 ½ cups semi skimmed milk

2 free range eggs, beaten
1 tsp low fat 'butter' spread
½ tsp paprika
½ tsp ground nutmeg

Method:

Combine all the ingredients, except the nutmeg, in the slow cooker. Cover and leave to cook on low for 3-4 hours or high for 2-3 hours. Make sure the pasta is tender. Add more milk if needed and stir well. Sprinkle with nutmeg before serving.

Using the evaporated milk in this recipe makes for a lovely, creamy consistency. Mare sure you don't overcook the macaroni.

Pomodoro Pasta Sauce
Serves 4

Ingredients:

2 400g/14oz tins chopped tomatoes

6 large fresh tomatoes, chopped (vine ripened are best)

250ml/1 cup tomato passata/ sieved tomatoes

Handful sliced black olives

120ml/ ½ cup vegetable stock/ broth

3 tbsp freshly chopped basil

3 garlic cloves, crushed

1 onion, chopped

1 tsp brown sugar

1 tsp extra virgin olive oil

Salt and pepper to taste

Method:

Combine all the ingredients in the slow cooker. Season, cover and leave to cook on low for 6-8 hours or high 3-4 hours. Delicious served with angel hair pasta, salad & grated vegetarian parmesan style cheese.

This is a classic tomato based Italian pasta sauce which gets better the long you leave it. Reheated leftovers seem to have a greater depth of taste which is worth waiting for.

Risi e Bisi
Serves 4

Ingredients:

300g/11oz long grain rice
250ml/1 cup vegetable stock/broth
1 carrot, finely chopped
1 large onion, finely chopped
3 cloves garlic, crushed
75g/3oz french beans, sliced
150g/5oz frozen peas

1 tsp each rosemary, basil & thyme
Handful pitted olives, chopped
1 tbsp freshly grated lemon zest
75g/3ozl ripe cherry tomatoes, chopped
1 tbsp lemon juice
Salt & pepper to taste

Method:

Combine all the ingredients, except the lemon juice, in the slow cooker. Season, cover and leave to cook on high for 2-3 hours with the lid tightly shut. The rice may need a little more stock during cooking. Make sure it is tender, stir through the lemon juice and serve with a grated vegetarian hard cheese, rocket and avocado slices.

Translated simply as 'Rice & Peas', this recipe really benefits from a squeeze of lemon before serving.

Bean, Potato & Cheese Stew
Serves 4

385 CALORIES PER SERVING

Ingredients:

1 400g/14oz tin sweetcorn
1 400g/14oz tin mixed beans
1 red (bell) pepper, chopped
1 large onion, chopped
500ml/2 cups tomato passata/
sieved tomatoes

1 tsp each cumin and coriander
75g/3oz grated cheddar cheese
150g/5oz potatoes, diced
½ tsp cayenne pepper
Juice of one lemon
Salt & pepper to taste

Method:

Add all the ingredients to the slow cooker except the cheese.
Combine well and then sprinkle the cheese onto the top. Season,
cover and cook on low for 5-6 hours or on high for 3-4 hours.
Make sure the potatoes are cooked right through and serve with
sour cream and flat bread. If you find the stew is a little dry during
cooking add some water to loosen.

*This vegetarian meal is a lovely Mexican inspired dish.
Feel free to spice it up with extra cayenne pepper if
you like and serve with an onion & tomato or green
salad.*

Apple Root Stew
Serves 4

165
CALORIES
PER SERVING

Ingredients:

1 parsnip, chopped
3 carrots, chopped
100g/3 ½ oz sweet potato, cubed
1 onion, chopped
100g/3 ½ oz turnip, cubed

3 tbsp balsamic vinegar
1 garlic clove, crushed
1 tbsp olive oil
Salt & pepper to taste
250ml/1 cup apple juice

Method:

Combine all the ingredients in the slow cooker. Season, cover and leave to cook on low for 6-8 hours or on high for 3-5 hours. You may need to add a little water during cooking. Make sure all the vegetables are tender and serve with chopped flat leaf parsley and crusty farmhouse bread.

You could use squash instead of sweet potato in this recipe if you prefer.

Berber Rice Baked Peppers

Serves 4

270 CALORIES PER SERVING

Ingredients:

4 large red, green or yellow (bell) peppers
1 400g/14oz tin butter beans, drained
125g/4oz vegetarian feta-style cheese
75g/3oz couscous
Bunch spring onions/scallions, chopped

2 garlic cloves, crushed
1 tsp each dried oregano and basil
75g/3oz frozen peas
120ml/ ½ cup water (more if needed during cooking)
Salt & pepper to taste
2 tbsp lemon juice

Method:

Take the tops off the peppers and scoop out the inside so you have an empty pepper shell. Combine together all the other ingredients (except lemon juice and water) and then stuff into each of the peppers. Sit the peppers upright in the slow cooker, pour the water around them, and leave to cook on high for 3-4 hours with the lid tightly closed. Add some lemon juice to the tops and serve with a dollop of Greek yoghurt.

The couscous (North African Berber rice) and Greek herbs in this dish are a great combination.

Double Potato Casserole

Serves 4

238 CALORIES PER SERVING

Ingredients:

450g/1lb desiree potatoes, cubed

300g/11oz sweet potatoes, cubed

2 carrots, cubed

2 parsnips, cubed

1 onion, chopped

2 celery sticks, chopped

1 400g/14oz tin condensed mushroom soup

2 garlic cloves, crushed

120ml/ ½ cup vegetable stock

½ tsp ground nutmeg

Method:

Place all the ingredients in the slow cooker and combine well. Cover, season and leave to cook on low for 4-6 hours or until the vegetables are tender. Add a little more stock during cooking if needed. Serve with steamed greens.

Using both sweet potatoes and desiree potatoes in this recipe creates a great combination.

Beetroot Bean Salad Topping

Serves 4

Ingredients:

1 onion, chopped

450g/1lb fresh raw beetroot, cubed

2 400g/14oz tins cannellini beans, drained

375ml/1½cups vegetable stock/broth

3 tbsp fresh chopped coriander/cilantro

Salt & pepper to taste

Method:

Gently sauté the onions in a little low cal spray for a few minutes until soft. Add all the ingredients to the slow cooker and gently combine. Cover, season and leave to cook on low for 3-5 hours or until everything is tender and cooked through. Add a little more stock during cooking if needed. Serve with green salad, red onions & Greek yoghurt.

Fresh beetroot is a much overlooked ingredient which, if given a chance, can form the heart of a good meal.

Spiced Sweet Potatoes & Eggs

Serves 4

Ingredients:

1 onion, chopped
1 tsp each ground cumin, coriander/cilantro & turmeric
½ tsp each chilli power, crushed chilli flakes & garam masala
1 400g/14oz tins chopped tomatoes
250ml/1 cup vegetable stock/ broth
300g/11oz sweet potatoes, peeled & cubed

4 free range eggs, hard-boiled, peeled and quartered
60ml/¼ cup single cream
3 garlic cloves, crushed
200g/7oz lentils, soaked overnight
1 tsp brown sugar
100g/3½ oz peas
100g/3½ oz baby sweetcorn
Low cal cooking spray
Salt & pepper to taste

Method:

Gently sauté the onions in a little low cal spray for a few minutes until soft. Add all the ingredients to the slow cooker, except the cream and eggs, and gently combine. Cover, season and leave to cook on low for 5-7 hours or until everything is tender and cooked through. 10 minutes before serving add the eggs and cream and gently stir through. Serve with rice or flat bread and salad.

If you prefer you can use your eggs in a different way by breaking them raw into the slow cooker half an hour before the end of cooking so that they set whole in the dish.

Kale & Lentil Supper
Serves 4

Ingredients:

200g/7oz kale, shredded
1 tsp olive oil
300g/11oz lentils
1 onion, chopped
4 garlic cloves, crushed
3 roasted red peppers, sliced
(shop bought)
1 400g/14oz tin chopped
tomatoes

½ tsp sea salt
1 tsp each, ginger, cumin &
coriander/cilantro
250ml/1 cups vegetable/stock
broth
Salt & pepper to taste

Method:

Add all the ingredients into the slow cooker. Season, cover and
leave to cook on low for 4-6 hours or until the lentils are tender
and the stock absorbed. Add a little more stock during cooking if
needed.

*Kale is a real super-food which has enjoyed a massive
surge in popularity in recent years. It can be a little
tough but slow cooking counteracts this beautifully.*

Creamed Cheese & Sweetcorn Supper

Serves 4

Ingredients:

750g/1lb 9oz frozen sweetcorn
1 400g/14oz tin creamed
sweetcorn
200g/7oz low fat cream cheese
1 tbsp brown sugar

125g/4oz cheddar cheese,
grated
4 tbsp water
Salt & pepper to taste

Method:

Add all the ingredients to the slow cooker. Combine well, season, cover and leave to cook on low for 3-5 hours or until everything is cooked through and tender. Add a little more water during cooking if needed. Alternatively if you want to thicken things up a little, remove the lid and leave to cook on high for aprox 45 minutes longer or until you achieve the desired consistency.

Serve with sliced seasoned tomatoes & rocket salad.

This is the food of good childhood memories. It's almost pudding-like in it's consistency and invariably popular with the whole family.

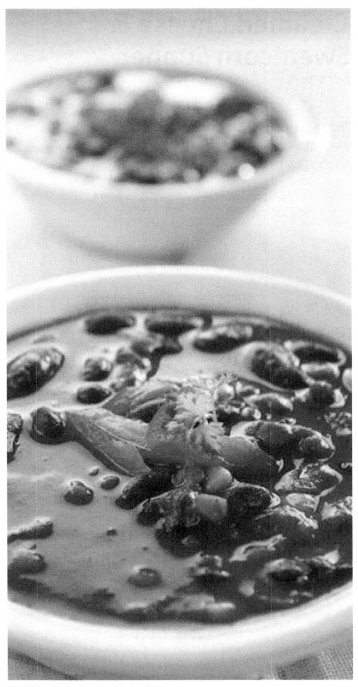

Capsicum Mexican Chilli

Serves 4

Ingredients:

1 400g/14oz tin chopped tomatoes

1 200g/7oz tin kidney beans. drained

1 200g/7oz tin chickpeas, drained

1 200g/ 7oz tin sweetcorn

1 courgette/zucchini sliced

1 onion, chopped

1 carrot, sliced

1 stalk celery, sliced

1 tsp chilli powder (or to taste)

1 tsp paprika

2 cloves garlic, crushed

500ml/2 cups vegetable stock/ broth

3 tbsp tomato puree/paste

1 tbsp balsamic vinegar

1 tsp dried oregano

2 tsp ground cumin

1 whole bay leaf

1 tsp salt

Method:

Combine all ingredients in the slow cooker, cover and leave to cook on low for 5-6 or high for 3 to 4 hours. Add a little more stock during cooking if needed, or if it needs thickening remove the lid and leave to cook on high for a further 45 minutes or until you get the desired consistency.

Remove the bay leaf; serve with rice and soured cream.

You can alter this recipe to include whichever beans you have to hand and feel free to fine tune the chilli powder to your own taste.

Lemon & Hazelnut Broccoli

Serves 4

Ingredients:

900g/2lb broccoli florets
2 tbsp olive oil
6 tbsp lemon juice
½ tsp sea salt

2 tbsp water
125g/4oz hazelnuts, chopped
6 cloves garlic, crushed
Salt & pepper to taste

Method:

Add all the ingredients to the slow cooker. Combine well, season, cover and leave to cook on high for 2-3 hours or until the broccoli is tender, but not overcooked. Add a little more water during cooking if needed. Serve with soy-soaked noodles and a pinch of chilli flakes.

If you prefer more crunch, add the hazelnuts at the very end of the cooking time rather than the beginning.

Garlic & Broccoli Breadcrumb Pasta

Serves 4

Ingredients:

300g/11oz fusilli pasta
600g/1lb 5oz tenderstem
broccoli, chopped
3 cloves garlic, crushed
1 tsp olive oil
60ml/¼ cup vegetable stock

¼ tsp crushed chilli flakes (or
more to taste)
1 slice bread
3 tbsp lemon juice
Salt & pepper to taste

Method:

Place the broccoli, garlic, lemon juice and stock in the slow cooker and combine well. Cover, season and leave to cook on high for 1-3 hours or until tender.

Meanwhile cook the pasta in salted boiling water until tender, then drain. Place the bread in a food processor and whizz to make breadcrumbs. Heat the oil in a frying pan and fry the breadcrumbs until crispy.

Combine the cooked broccoli and pasta together. Season well, sprinkle with the breadcrumbs and serve.

You could also add some lemon zest to the breadcrumbs when they are frying for extra 'zing'!

Sweet Beans & Spinach
Serves 4

Ingredients:

375g/13oz spinach leaves,
1 400g/14oz tins borlotti beans, drained
1 400g/14oz tin black beans, drained
1 onion, chopped
100g/3½oz sweet potatoes, chopped
3 cloves garlic, crushed
1 tsp each cumin, turmeric & coriander/cilantro
½ tsp sea salt
3 tbsp lemon juice
60ml/½cup runny honey
60ml/½cup vegetable stock/broth
2 tbsp low fat cream cheese

Method:

Add all the ingredients to the slow cooker. Combine well, season, cover and leave to cook on low for 5-6 hours or high for 3-4 hours or until everything is cooked through and tender. Add a little more stock during cooking if needed. Alternatively if you want to thicken things up a little, remove the lid and leave to cook on high for aprox 45 minutes longer or until you achieve the desired consistency.

This sweet dish is super filling and is lovely eaten cold too.

Vegetarian Sausage & Spinach With Gnocchi

Serves 4

Ingredients:

6 vegetarian sausages
250ml/1 cup passata/sieved tomatoes
1 tsp dried rosemary

1 splash red wine vinegar
½ tsp salt
100g/3½oz fresh spinach
500g/1lb 2oz gnocchi

Method:

Brown the sausages in a frying pan and cut into pieces. Add all the ingredients, except the gnocchi and spinach, to the slow cooker and combine well. Close the lid tightly and leave to cook on low for 5-6 hours or high for 3-4 hours. Stir in the spinach and gnocchi and leave to cook for a further 10 mins or until the gnocchi is tender.

Add a little sugar to this recipe if the tomatoes and vinegar are a little sharp.

Basil, Peppers & Gnocchi
Serves 4

Ingredients:

1 onion, chopped
3 yellow peppers, sliced
1 400g/14oz tin chopped tomatoes
2 cloves of garlic
1 tsp brown sugar
4 tbsp freshly chopped basil

120ml/½ cup vegetable stock/broth
500g/1lb 2oz gnocchi
Salt & pepper to taste
1 tbsp grated vegetarian parmesan-style cheese
Low cal cooking spray

Method:

Gently sauté the peppers and onion in a little low cal cooking spray. Add all the ingredients, except the gnocchi and cheese, to the slow cooker and combine well. Season, cover and leave to cook on low for 5-6 hours or high for 3-4 hours. Stir in the gnocchi and leave to cook for a further 10 mins or until the gnocchi is tender. Sprinkle the cheese on top and serve.

Shop bought roasted peppers are also lovely in place of the fresh ones used here.

Mushroom Ragu
Serves 4

Ingredients:

2 garlic cloves, crushed
900g/2lb mixed mushrooms
3 tbsp port wine
1 400g/14oz tin chopped tomatoes
2 tbsp balsamic vinegar

3 tbsp freshly chopped basil
3 tbsp freshly chopped flat leaf parsley
1 tsp brown sugar
Low cal cooking spray
Salt & pepper to taste

Method:

Gently sauté the mushrooms, onion and garlic in a little low cal cooking spray for a few minutes. Add all the ingredients to the slow cooker and combine well. Season, cover and leave to cook on low for 5-6 hours or high for 3-4 hours. Serve with crusty bread.

Feel free to increase the port and balsamic vinegar quantities in this recipe if you prefer.

43

Basil Zucchini Bake
Serves 4

190 CALORIES PER SERVING

Ingredients:

700g/1lb 9oz courgette/
zucchini, cubed
1 200g/7oz tin condensed
mushroom soup
1 onion, chopped
2 carrots, chopped

1 tbsp olive oil
120ml/½ cup vegetable stock
250g/9oz broad beans
3 tbsp freshly chopped basil
2 garlic cloves, crushed
Salt & pepper to taste

Method:

Place all the ingredients in the slow cooker and combine well.
Cover, season and leave to cook on low for 4-6 hours or until the
vegetables are tender. Add a little more stock during cooking if
needed.

*Try reducing the cooking time on this recipe if you
prefer your courgettes a little crunchy.*

Paprika Potatoes
Serves 4

Ingredients:

1 red onion, sliced
1 tsp each paprika & smoked paprika
2 red (bell) peppers, sliced
1 400g/14oz tin chopped tomatoes
120ml/½ cup vegetable stock/broth
1 tsp rock salt
½ tsp brown sugar
600g/1lb 5oz potatoes, cubed
1 tsp each rosemary & thyme
50g/2oz black pitted olives, chopped
Low cal cooking spray

Method:

Gently sauté the onions in a little low cal spray for a few minutes until soft. Add all the ingredients to the slow cooker, except the olives. Cover and leave to cook on high for 3-5 hours or until everything is tender and cooked through. 30 minutes before serving add the olives and gently warm through.

If there is too much liquid, continue to cook on high with the lid off for aprox 45 minutes or until you achieve the consistency you prefer.

Using smoked paprika in this recipe is great but you could also add a little fire to that smokiness with some cayenne pepper if you like.

Tomato & Garlic Mushrooms

Serves 4

Ingredients:

1 tbsp olive oil
450g/1lb chestnut mushrooms
5 cloves garlic, crushed
1 stick celery
1 400g/14oz tin chopped
tomatoes

1 tbsp tomato puree/paste
3 tbsp fresh chopped flat leaf
parsley
½ tsp crushed chilli flakes
1 onion, chopped

Method:

Add all the ingredients to the slow cooker, except the parsley.
Season, cover and leave to cook on high for 3-4 hours or low for
5-6 hours or until the mushrooms are tender and the flavours
have thoroughly blended.

*This is great served with spaghetti & salad for a
delicious Italian meal, or on bruschetta as a snack.*

Fennel Risotto
Serves 4

Ingredients:

1 fennel bulb, diced
250g/9oz risotto rice
1 carrot, chopped
1 onion, chopped
25g/1oz grated parmesan
cheese
50g/2oz black olives, finely
chopped

3 garlic cloves, crushed
1lt/4 cups vegetable stock/
broth
125g/4oz frozen peas
50g/2oz rocket
15g/ ½ oz butter
Salt & pepper to taste

Method:

Preheat the slow cooker and place the butter in the bottom. When it is melted, add the risotto rice and stir well until every grain is finely coated. Add the rest of the ingredients, except the cheese and rocket, to the slow cooker and season well. Cover and leave to cook on high for 2-3 hours. If you need to add more liquid during cooking go ahead by adding just a little each time. After cooking, all the liquid should be absorbed and the rice should be tender. If it isn't, leave to cook for a little longer with the lid off. Serve sprinkled with parmesan cheese and the rocket piled on top.

Risotto usually needs a lot of stirring during cooking. This slow cooker alternative is a great labour saver with virtually no stirring required.

Boston Bean Dream

Serves 4

Ingredients:

1 tsp groundnut or vegetable oil

1 red onion, sliced into rounds

1 tbsp brown sugar

1 400g/14oz tin chopped tomatoes

250ml/1 cup vegetable stock/ broth

1 400g/14oz tin cannellini beans, drained

1 400g/14oz tin butter beans, drained

50g/2oz sweetcorn

2 tbsp dijon mustard

1 tsp paprika

Salt & pepper to taste

Method:

Gently sauté the onions in a frying pan with the oil for a few minutes. Combine all the ingredients into the slow cooker, season, cover and leave to cook on low for 4-6 hours or on high for 2-3 hours. Add a little more stock during cooking if needed, or if it needs thickening remove the lid and leave to cook on high for a further 45 minutes or until you get the desired consistency. Serve with a dollop of sour cream and some flat bread.

Vine ripened or fresh cherry tomatoes will work even better than the tinned variety.

48

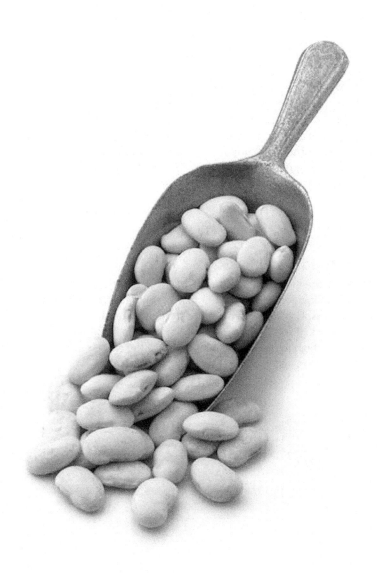

Lentil Dhal
Serves 4

Ingredients:

400g/14oz split red lentils
1 onion, chopped
1 garlic clove, crushed
1 tsp each ground coriander/
cilantro, turmeric & cumin
½ each tsp ground ginger,
paprika & mustard seeds

500ml/2 cups vegetable stock/
broth
2 tbsp freshly chopped
coriander/cilantro
25g/1oz butter
Salt & pepper to taste

Method:

Add all the ingredients to the slow cooker, cover and leave to cook on low for 4-6 hours or until the lentils are tender and the liquid absorbed. Add a little more stock or water during cooking if needed. If there is too much liquid, take the lid off and leave to cook on high for approx 40 mins. Sprinkle the chopped coriander over the top and serve.

Dhal is a one of the most common dishes in Asia. It is eaten by some families at almost every single meal time. This simple version is great served with Indian chapatti bread.

50

Butter Beans & Almond Stew

Serves 4

206 CALORIES PER SERVING

Ingredients:

1 onion, sliced into rounds
2 garlic cloves, crushed
300g/11oz new potatoes, sliced
1 tsp mustard seeds
2 tbsp tomato puree/paste
½ tsp ground cinnamon
1 celery stick, chopped
450g/1lb cauliflower florets
50g/2oz sultanas

200g/7oz tinned butter beans, drained
50g/2oz chopped almonds
1 400g/14oz tin chopped tomatoes
250ml/1 cup vegetable stock/broth
Salt & pepper to taste

Method:

Add all the ingredients to the slow cooker, cover, stir well and leave to cook on high for 2-3 hours or low for 4-5 hours or until the vegetables are tender.

If you want the stew a little thicker, take the lid off and continue to cook on high for 45mins or until the consistency is to your liking.

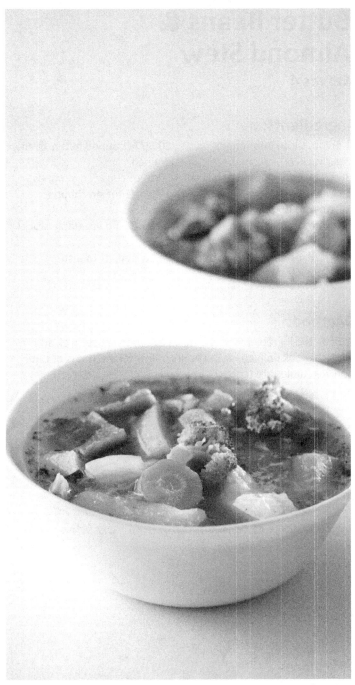

THE Skinny SLOW COOKER VEGETARIAN
RECIPE BOOK

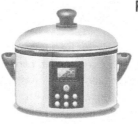

SOUPS

Corn & Potato Chowder

Serves 4

Ingredients:

1 onion, chopped
2 400g/14oz tins sweetcorn, drained
1 400g/14oz tin creamed sweetcorn
2 cloves garlic, crushed

750ml/3 cups vegetable stock
250g/9oz potatoes, diced
1 tsp low fat 'butter' spread
500ml/2 cups semi skimmed milk
1 tsp salt

Method:

Sauté the onion and garlic in the 'butter'. Place all the ingredients in the slow cooker, cover, season and cook on low for 3-4 hours. Ensure the potatoes are tender and mash a little with a fork to create the right consistency. Serve with saltine or cream crackers for an authentic finish.

Although primarily associated with seafood, chowder is a lovely thick soup recipe which works just as well with vegetables alone.

Barley & Chestnut Mushroom Soup

Serves 4

Ingredients:

1 large onion, chopped
1 tsp olive oil
1 carrot, chopped
1 celery stalk, chopped
200g/7oz mushrooms, finely chopped
1 400g/14oz tin chopped tomatoes

200g/7oz frozen sweetcorn
100g/3 ½ oz pearl barley
1 tsp each of basil, oregano, thyme
Salt & pepper to taste
3 cloves garlic, crushed
1 lt/4 cups vegetable stock

Method:

Gently sauté the onions, carrot, mushrooms and celery in a frying pan with the olive oil for a few minutes. Combine all the ingredients into the slow cooker, season, cover and leave to cook on low for 4-5 hours or on for high 2-3 hours or until the barley is tender.

You could also introduce some spinach to this recipe which you add a minute or two before serving so that it is gently wilted.

This is a really tasty and filling soup. The mushrooms should be finely chopped to give the liquid of the soup some 'body'.

55

St. Patrick's Day Soup

Serves 4

Ingredients:

300g/11oz potatoes, chopped
1 large onion, chopped
2 leeks, chopped
500ml/2 cups skimmed milk

500ml/2 cups vegetable stock/
broth
Salt & pepper to taste

Method:

Combine all the ingredients together in the slow cooker. Season, cover and leave to cook on low for 6-8 hours with the lid tightly shut. Make sure the potatoes are tender and then either blend as a smooth soup or eat it rough, ready and rustic with some crusty bread and a swirl of single cream.

It is often said that everyone is Irish on St. Patrick's Day. Here's a chance to get a real taste of Ireland every day with this lovely Irish inspired potato soup.

Asian Hot Soup
Serves 4

Ingredients:

75g/3oz shiitake mushrooms
50g/2 oz cloud ear fungus (or similar)
200g/7oz tinned bamboo shoots, drained
3 cloves garlic, crushed
1 tsp sesame oil
1 tsp dried crushed chillies
2 tbsp rice wine vinegar or wine vinegar

225g/8oz frozen peas
2 tbsp soy sauce
1 tsp sesame oil
275g/10oz tofu, cubed
1 tbsp freshly grated ginger
750ml/3 cups vegetable stock/ broth
Salt & pepper to taste

Method:

Combine all the ingredients in the slow cooker. Season, cover and leave to cook on low 4-6 hours or high for 2-3 hours. Serve with fresh chopped coriander/cilantro.

Chinese Hot & Sour soup is believed to be good for colds, so feel free to load up on the fresh ginger if you can handle it.

Zucchini Soup
Serves 4

Ingredients:

75g/3oz potato, cubed
750ml/3 cups vegetable stock/
broth
1 head broccoli, chopped
1 head cauliflower, chopped
1 tsp each cumin and paprika

Salt & pepper to taste
1 tsp olive oil
1 onion
2 garlic cloves, crushed
3 courgettes/zucchinis,
chopped

Method:

Gently sauté the onion and courgettes/zucchinis in the oil for a
few minutes. Add all the ingredients into the slow cooker. Cover,
season and leave to cook on low for 4-6 hours or high for 2-3
hours. Serve pureed or chunky with a swirl of fresh cream and a
sprinkle of grated parmesan style vegetarian cheese.

*You can mix this soup up by switching the broccoli
and courgette/zucchini measurements during cooking
and adding a little crumbled vegetarian stilton before
serving.*

Squash, Basil & Tomato Soup

Serves 4

Ingredients:

400g/14oz butternut squash
flesh, cubed
75g/3oz potatoes, peeled &
cubed
8 fresh vine tomatoes, chopped
½ tsp sugar
2 tbsp freshly chopped basil
leaves

4 tbsp tomato puree/paste
1lt/4 cups vegetable stock/
broth
60ml/¼ cup single cream
Salt & pepper to taste

Method:

Place all the ingredients, except the cream, in the slow cooker.
Season, cover and leave to cook on low for 3-4 hours or until the
vegetables are tender. After cooking blend the soup to a smooth
consistency and serve with a swirl of fresh cream.

*Butternut squash is a perfect slow cooker ingredient.
Its creamy, firm texture holds well during cooking and
forms a robust base to this tasty soup.*

Spicy Carrot Soup
Serves 4

Ingredients:

2 tsp ground cumin
½ tsp crushed chilli flakes
1 tbsp olive oil
750g/1lb 11oz carrots, finely chopped
½ onion, finely chopped

140g/4 ½ oz split red lentils
750ml/3 cups vegetable stock/broth
120ml/ ½ cup milk
60ml/ ¼ cup single cream
Salt & pepper to taste.

Method:

Add all the ingredients to the slow cooker, except the cream and milk. Season, cover and leave to cook on high for aprox 3 hours or until the lentils are tender. Add the milk and warm through for a minute or two. Use a food processor or blender to whizz the soup to a smooth consistency and serve with a swirl of single cream in each bowl.

This warming soup can be tweaked to suit your taste - add more or less chilli flakes as you prefer. Plus if you want to reduce the calories a little, swap the olive oil for low cal cooking spray and the regular milk for skimmed.

Flagelot & Savoy Soup

Serves 4

Ingredients:

1 onion, finely chopped
1 carrot, finely chopped
1 whole savoy cabbage, chopped
1 tbsp olive oil
1lt/4 cups vegetable stock/broth

2 tbsp tomato puree/paste
1 tsp each dried oregano & rosemary
Salt & pepper to taste
1 400g/14oz tin flagolet beans, drained

Method:

Place all the ingredients in the slow cooker. Season, cover and leave to cook on low for 3-4 hours or until the vegetables are tender. Adjust the seasoning and serve.

This soup is best served chunky. If however, you prefer a smoother consistency, reserve a ladle of flageolet beans from the cooked soup, blend the rest of the soup and stir the whole beans back through before stirring.

Parsnip & Coconut Milk Soup

Serves 4

140 CALORIES PER SERVING

Ingredients:

1 onion, chopped
4 parsnips, chopped
4 carrots, chopped
1 tsp each turmeric, cumin, coriander/cilantro & paprika
120ml/1 cup low fat coconut milk

2 tbsp freshly chopped chives
750ml/3 cups vegetable stock/broth
Salt & pepper to taste
250ml/1 cup fat free Greek yoghurt

Method:

Place all the ingredients, except the chives, coconut milk & yoghurt in the slow cooker. Season, cover and leave to cook on low for 3-4 hours or until the vegetables are tender. After cooking, blend the soup to a smooth consistency and serve with a dollop of yoghurt in the middle and some fresh chives sprinkled on top.

Adding the coconut milk during lengthy cooking risks the milk 'splitting', so leave it until the end and warm through.

Spinach & Haricot Soup

Serves 6

Ingredients:

2 lt/8 cups vegetable stock/broth
4 tbsp tomato puree/paste
1 400g/14oz tin haricot beans, rinsed
250g/9oz brown rice

200g/7oz spinach
2 onions, chopped
2 garlic cloves, crushed
1 tsp each dried basil & oregano
Salt & pepper to taste

Method:

Combine all the ingredients, except the spinach, into the slow cooker. Season, cover and leave to cook on low for 5-6 hours or high for 3-4 hours. 20 minutes before the end of cooking, stir through the spinach. Serve with crusty bread.

This hearty soup is great freshened up with a twist of lemon and chopped basil to garnish.

THE
Skinny SLOW
COOKER
VEGETARIAN
RECIPE BOOK

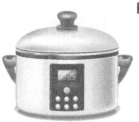

APPETISERS/SNACKS

Sweet & Salty Almond Snack or Killer Salad!
Serves 5-6

Ingredients:

1lb / 250g almonds
75g/3oz brown sugar
½ tsp each cayenne pepper,
cumin, cinnamon & nutmeg
2 tbsp reduced sugar honey

2 tbsp sugar free maple syrup
2 tbsp low fat 'butter' spread
1½ tsp crushed sea salt flakes
60ml/ ¼ cup water

Method:

Combine all the ingredients into the slow cooker and leave to cook on low for 4-6 hours with the lid tightly shut. Ensure the nuts do not burn; add a little more water during cooking if needed.

Calories stated are per 50g serving.

This is a delicious and indulgent snack which can also be served as the topping for a killer salad. You can use whichever nut you prefer, the recipe here uses whole almonds but any whole nut will work equally well.

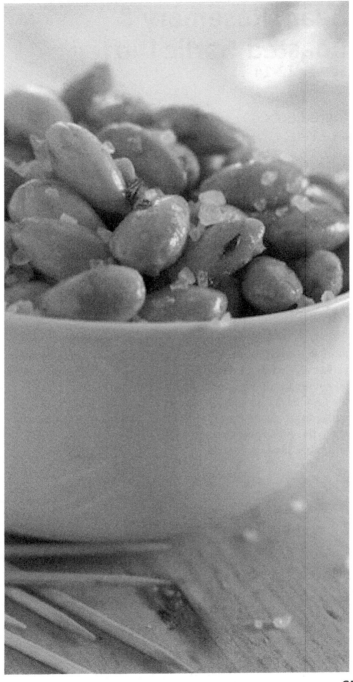

Bean, Rosemary & Roasted Garlic Dip

Serves 12-14

Ingredients:

6 garlic cloves, chopped
100g/3 ½ oz vegetarian parmesan-style cheese grated
3 tbsp chopped fresh rosemary
2 tbsp extra virgin olive oil
1 400g/14oz tin borlotti beans, drained

125g/4oz low fat vegetarian cream cheese
Handful chopped black olives
1 tbsp white wine vinegar
1 cup/250ml water
1 tbsp lemon juice
Salt & pepper to taste

Method:

Quickly pulse together all the ingredients (except the lemon juice) in a food processor. Empty the blitzed mixture into the slow cooker and leave to cook on low for 1-2 hours. The dip may need a little more water during cooking, or if it needs thickening remove the lid and leave to cook on high for a further 45 minutes or until you get the desired consistency. After cooking allow to cool, stir in the lemon juice and serve with a selection of raw celery, cucumber and carrot batons.

This is a perfect low cal snack to keep you going between meals.

Italian Mushrooms
Serves 4

Ingredients:

3 tbsp extra-virgin olive oil
450g/1lb chestnut or portobella mushrooms
250g/9oz vegetarian ricotta cheese
2 tbsp vegetarian green pesto + 1 extra for serving

2 garlic cloves, crushed
25g/1 oz grated vegetarian parmesan-style cheese
120ml/ ½ cup vegetable stock/ broth
Salt & pepper to taste

Method:

Combine all the ingredients (except the cheese and 1 tbsp pesto) in the slow cooker. Cover, season and leave to cook on low for 4-6 hours . The mushrooms may need a little more water during cooking, or if it needs thickening remove the lid and leave to cook on high for a further 45 minutes or until you get the desired consistency. Drain any excess liquid off and add the extra pesto and grated cheese on top.

Serve with pitta bread and salad or over pasta.

Red pesto as an alternative to green pesto gives an altogether different taste to this recipe.

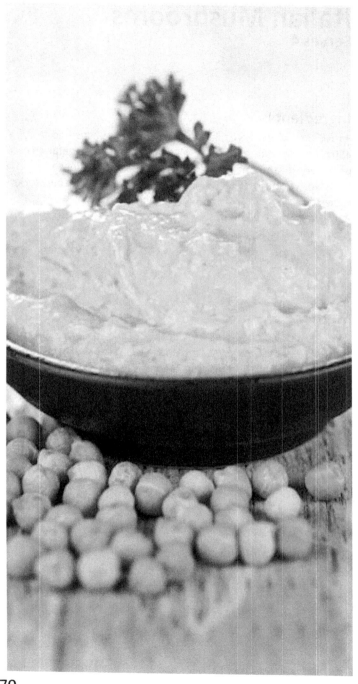

Hummus bi tahini
Serves 8

Ingredients:

400g/14oz tinned chickpeas,
drained
6 cloves garlic, crushed
4 tbsp lemon juice

1 tbsp salt
2 tbsp olive oil
120ml/ ½ cup water
3 tbsp tahini

Method:

Add the chickpeas to the slow cooker and cover well with water.
Cook on low with the lid tightly shut for 6-8 hours. Add a little
more water if needed and cook until completely tender.   Scoop
out your chickpeas and combine with all the other ingredients in a
food processor. Blend until it's a smooth as you prefer, using some
of the leftover chickpea liquid still in the slow cooker to get the
consistency you want.

*Arabic for 'chickpeas with tahini' - humous (hummus)
is an ancient food which has been enjoyed for more
than a millennia. This is a really inexpensive way of
making up a good batch. You can make your own
versions by adding chopped sundried tomatoes or
olives.*

Braised Garlic Sauerkraut

Serves 4

Ingredients:

1 head green cabbage, chopped
1 large onion, chopped
200g/7oz tinned chopped tomatoes
200g/7oz tinned sauerkraut

2 garlic cloves, crushed
½ tsp celery salt
25g/1oz low fat 'butter' spread
2 tbsp brown sugar
Salt & pepper to taste

Method:

Add all the ingredients to the slow cooker. Combine well, season, cover and leave to cook on low for 4-6 hours or until everything is cooked through and tender. Add a little water during cooking if needed.

You can easily increase the garlic in this recipe by adding some whole cloves if you want to make it really garlickly.

Slow Cooked Corn
Serves 4

Ingredients:

4 large cobs of corn, husks left
on
2 tbsp water

Method:

Add the water and corn to the slow cooker. Cover and leave to
cook on low 2-3 hours or until tender. Add a little more water
during cooking if needed. Peel the husks off the corn and if you
like, serve with garlic oil.

*When the corn is cooked you could sprinkle a little
paprika or cayenne pepper over the top before serving
to give a little 'kick'.*

Spiced Creamed Spinach
Serves 4

95 CALORIES PER SERVING

Ingredients:

600g/1lb 5oz spinach
1 tsp olive oil
1 onion, chopped
2 garlic cloves, crushed
1 tsp crushed chilli flakes

3 fresh tomatoes, chopped
3 tbsp water
4 tablespoons fat- free crème fraiche
Salt & pepper to taste

Method:

Place all the ingredients, except the crème fraiche, in the slow cooker. Cover, season and leave to cook on low for 3-5 hours. Add a little more water during cooking if needed. Stir through the crème fraiche and serve.

Some finely chopped spring onions/scallions provide a nice garnish to this creamy side dish.

Apple Sauce
Serves 4

Ingredients:

4 large cooking apples, peeled
& cored
2 tbsp lemon juice
1 tsp vanilla extract

60ml/¼ cup water
1 tsp brown sugar
½ tsp ground cinnamon

Method:

Place all the ingredients in the slow cooker. Cover and leave to cook on low for 3-5 hours. Add a little more water during cooking if needed and pulp with the back of a fork. Alternatively if you want to thicken things up, remove the lid and leave to cook on high for aprox 45 minutes longer or until you achieve the desired consistency.

Homemade apple sauce is a completely different beast to the shop-bought version. Increase the cinnamon if you want it to be even more aromatic.

Nacho Bean & Onion Dip

Serves 4

Ingredients:

2 400g/14oz tins low fat refried beans
1 green chilli, finely chopped
1 large onion, chopped
100g/3 ½ oz mozzarella cheese, chopped
1 packet of your favourite taco seasoning mix
Salt to taste
250ml/1 cup water
1 tbsp lemon juice

Or make your own taco mix:
2 tsp mild chilli powder, 1 ½ tsp ground cumin, ½ tsp paprika, ¼ tsp each of onion powder, garlic powder, dried oregano & crushed chilli flakes + 1 tsp each of sea salt & black pepper.

Method:

Place all the ingredients, except the lemon juice, into the slow cooker and combine well. Cover and leave to cook on low for 1-2 hours. The dip may need a little more water during cooking, or if it needs thickening remove the lid and leave to cook on high for a further 45 minutes or until you get the desired consistency. Before serving stir in the lemon juice. Serve warm with plain tortilla chips.

Buffallo mozzarello is good in this recipe but regular mozarella is fine too. Use the full fat versions of both.

Spiced Red Cabbage & Apple
Serves 4

Ingredients:

1 head red cabbage, cored and sliced
1 red onion, sliced
250ml/1 cup cider (sweet or dry is fine)
1 cooking apple, chopped

3 tbsp balsamic vinegar
1 tbsp brown sugar
½ tsp each ground ginger, cinnamon
¼ tsp nutmeg
Salt & pepper to taste

Method:

Add all the ingredients to the slow cooker. Combine well, season, cover and leave to cook on low for 4-6 hours or until everything is cooked through and tender. Add a little water during cooking if needed. Alternatively if you want to thicken things up, remove the lid and leave to cook on high for aprox 45 minutes longer or until you achieve the desired consistency.

The cider and vinegar in this recipe give the cabbage a nice bite and makes it a significant side dish.

Succotash
Serves 6

Ingredients:

200g/7oz sweetcorn
200g/7oz lima or kidney beans
200g/7oz creamed sweetcorn
1 red (bell) pepper, chopped
½ onion, chopped

½ tsp ground cumin
50g/2oz smoked gouda cheese
5 tbsp water
250ml/1 cup sour cream

Method:

Place all the ingredients, except the sour cream, in the slow cooker. Cover and leave to cook on low for 3-5 hours. Add a little more water during cooked if needed. Alternatively if you want to thicken things up, remove the lid and leave to cook on high for aprox 45 minutes longer or until you achieve the desired consistency. Remove from the heat and stir through the sour cream.

Lima beans are best in this traditional side dish but kidney beans will do fine.

Parmesan Style Green Beans
Serves 4

Ingredients:

250g/9oz green beans
1 red (bell) pepper, sliced
2 tsp low fat 'butter' spread
2 tbsp grated vegetarian parmesan-style cheese

½ tsp garlic salt
1 red onion, sliced
Salt & pepper to taste

Method:

Place all the ingredients in the slow cooker. Cover and leave to cook on low for 3-5 hours. Add a little water during cooked if needed.

Any strong vegetarian hard cheese will work just as well with this recipe.

Sweet & Sour Savoy
Serves 4

95 CALORIES PER SERVING

Ingredients:

2 tbsp brown sugar
1 tbsp plain/all purpose flour
1 tsp salt
120ml/½ cup water
60ml/¼ cup cider or wine vinegar

1 whole savoy cabbage, cored and shredded
1 onion, chopped

Method:

Place all the ingredients in the slow cooker and combine well. Cover and leave to cook on low for 3-5 hours. Add a little more water during cooked if needed.

Reduce the sugar in this recipe if you want to reduce the calories even more.

Silky Leeks & Peas
Serves 4

206 CALORIES PER SERVING

Ingredients:

4 leeks, sliced
25g/1oz low fat 'butter' spread
2 tbsp olive oil
250ml/1 cup vegetable stock/broth

500g/1lb2oz frozen peas
4 spring onions/scallions, sliced
2 garlic cloves, crushed
Salt & pepper to taste

Method:

Place all the ingredients in the slow cooker and combine well. Cover and leave to cook on low for 2-4 hours. Add a little more stock during cooked if needed.

A little single cream stirred through just before serving would make this dish even more silky.

Creamy Celery & Walnuts

Serves 4

Ingredients:

2 whole celery heads, trimmed and chopped
50g/2oz low fat 'butter' spread
1 onion, chopped
2 bay leaves
50g/2oz walnuts, chopped
75ml white wine

120ml/½ cup vegetable stock/broth
120ml/½ cup double cream
Salt & pepper to taste

Method:

Place all the ingredients, except the cream and walnuts, in the slow cooker and combine well. Cover and leave to cook on low for 2-4 hours. Add a little more stock during cooking if needed. Stir through the cream until warmed, sprinkle the walnuts over the top and serve.

You could cook the walnuts in this recipe by adding at the beginning of cooking if you want a soft nutty texture rather than adding at the end.

Marmalade Carrots
Serves 4

Ingredients:

700g/1lb 9oz baby carrots
100g/3 ½ oz marmalade
3 tbsp water

1 tbsp brown sugar
½ tsp ground cinnamon
Salt & pepper to taste

Method:

Place all the ingredients in the slow cooker and combine well. Cover, season and leave to cook on low for 2-4 hours or until the carrots are tender. Add a little more water during cooking if needed.

Traditional chunky orange marmalade is great, but lime marmalade works nicely too.

83

Honey Roasted Vegetables

Serves 4

Ingredients:

250g/9oz carrots
250g/9oz parsnips
1 tbsp balsamic vinegar
3 tsp runny honey
2 red onions
2 red (bell) peppers
2 tbsp olive oil

1 tsp each ground cumin, paprika, & chilli powder
½ tsp ground cinnamon
200g/7oz tinned chopped tomatoes
Salt & pepper to taste

Method:

Peel and cut the carrots, parsnips, peppers and onions into chunks. Combine all the ingredients well in the slow cooker. Season, cover and leave to cook on low for 3-4 hours or until the vegetables are tender. Add a little water during cooking if needed.

This is a great Moroccan inspired dish which is also nice with some chopped apricots if you like additional sweetness.

THE
Skinny SLOW
COOKER
VEGETARIAN
RECIPE BOOK

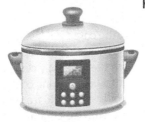

DESSERTS

Warming Spiced Apples
Serves 4

Ingredients:

4 medium cooking apples
125g/4oz raisins & sultanas
75g/3oz brown sugar
½ teaspoon each of nutmeg
and cinnamon

60ml/ ¼ cup apple juice
50g/2 oz chopped walnuts
1 tbsp low fat 'butter' spread

Method:

Core the apples. Mix together the raisins, brown sugar, spices and 'butter' then stuff into the cored apples. Add the apples to the slow cooker and pour the apple juice into the bottom. Leave to cook on a low heat with the lid tightly closed for 5-6 hours or high for 2-3 hours. Add a little water during cooking if needed. Remove the apples and spoon over any liquid from the bottom of the cooker. Delicious served with ice-cream.

This lovely dessert has a hint of Christmas spice to it which will warm you to the bone.

Cinnamon Apples
Serves 6

Ingredients:

6 cooking apples peeled, cored
and cut into wedges
1 tbsp lemon juice
75g/3oz brown sugar
75g/3oz raisins
75g/3oz chopped pecan nuts

125g/4oz low fat 'butter'
spread, gently melted
2 tsp ground cinnamon
120ml/ ½ cup water
1 tsp cornflour

Method:

Coat the apple slices well with the lemon juice and then combine
all the ingredients in the slow cooker. Cook on low for 3 hours
with the lid tightly shut or until the apples are tender. Add a little
more water during cooking if needed.

*The aroma around your home of the apple and
cinnamon as they cook is wonderful. This warming
dessert is even better served with a little cream or ice
cream on the side.*

Buckle Berry Cobbler
Serves 4

320 CALORIES PER SERVING

Ingredients:

75g/3oz plain/all purpose flour
200g/7oz brown sugar
½ tsp baking powder
½ tsp ground cinnamon
1 egg, lightly beaten

120ml/ ½ cup fat-free milk
2 tsp olive oil
150g/5oz raspberries
150g/5oz blueberries

Method:

Combine the flour, sugar, baking powder and cinnamon together. In a separate bowl mix together the egg, milk and oil. Gently combine both mixes together along with the fruit in the slow cooker and leave to cook on high for 2-3 hours with the lid tightly closed.

You can check the cobbler is ready by inserting a clean knife into the mixture. If it comes out clean it's cooked and ready to enjoy, if not leave it for a little longer.

Buckle cobbler is an old American term which means berries and batter. You can use any berries for this.

Bread Pudding
Serves 6

Ingredients:

5 slices cubed white bread (a
couple of days old is best)
500ml/2 cups skimmed milk
4 free range eggs
1 tsp ground cinnamon
100g/3 ½ oz brown sugar

125g/4oz low fat 'butter'
spread
½ tsp vanilla extract
¼ tsp ground nutmeg
150g/5oz raisins and sultanas

Method:

Combine all the ingredients in the slow cooker and leave to cook
on low for 3-5 hours with the lid tightly shut. The pudding may
need a little more milk during cooking, or if it needs thickening
remove the lid and leave to cook on high for a further 45 minutes
or until you get the desired consistency.

*This is a classic dessert recipe that everyone loves and
is so easy to make. If you are feeling indulgent you
could also add a handful of chocolate chips.*

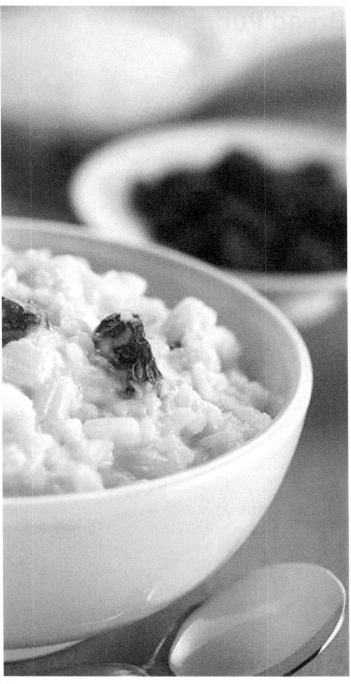

Rice pudding
Serves 4

Ingredients:

100g/3 ½oz pudding rice
½ tsp ground cinnamon
50g/2oz brown sugar
75g/3oz raisins or sultanas
750ml/3 cups semi skimmed milk

½ tsp ground nutmeg
1 bayleaf
1 tsp low fat 'butter' spread

Method:

Add the rice, sugar, butter, milk and bay leaf to the slow cooker and leave to cook on high for 2-3 hours with the lid tightly closed. Make sure the rice is nice and tender - you may need to add some milk during cooking if needed. Sprinkle over the nutmeg before serving and remove the bay leaf. Lovely served with a dollop of jam.

Rice pudding is a dish enjoyed by the people of almost every continent of the world. This European version was exported to the US by immigrants in the latter part of the 20th century.

Citrus Slice
Serves 6

Ingredients:

175g/6oz low fat 'butter' spread
100g/3 ½oz brown sugar
75g/3oz self raising flour
1 tbsp of lemon or lime zest
6 tbsp lemon or lime juice

3 egg yolks
120ml/ ½ cup semi skimmed milk
4 egg whites
250ml/1 cup water

Method:

Mix together the low fat spread and sugar, add the flour and lemon juice zest. Whisk in the egg yolks and milk.

Beat the egg whites until they peak then fold into your cake mixture. Pour the mixture into a cake tin and cover with foil. Add the water to the slow cooker and place the covered cake tin on top.

Cover and cook on low for 5-6 hours or until it is nicely cooked through. Serve with cream or ice cream as preferred.

This is a 'zingy' pudding, which although requires a little work, is well worth the effort.

Stewed Rhubarb & Cream

Serves 4

Ingredients:

500g/1lb 2oz rhubarb, chopped
100g/3½ oz brown sugar
3 tbsp water
250ml/1 cup single cream

Method:

Place all the ingredients, except the cream, in the slow cooker and combine well. Cover, season and leave to cook on low for 2-4 hours or until the rhubarb is very tender. Add a little more water during cooking if needed. Divide into bowls and swirl the cream over the top.

If you are lucky enough to have wild rhubarb growing locally, make use of the summer glut and freeze batches ready-stewed for later in the year.

Rum Bananas
Serves 4

Ingredients:

50g/2oz low fat 'butter' spread
3 tbsp brown sugar
6 bananas, thickly sliced
60ml/¼ cup rum

Method:

Place all the ingredients in the already warm slow cooker and gently combine until the 'butter' has melted. Cover and leave to cook for aprox 1hour on low. Delicious served with ice cream.

You could substitute madeira instead of the rum in this recipe if you wanted to try something different.

Apricots & Pistachios
Serves 4

Ingredients:

75g/3oz caster sugar
800g/1¾lb apricots, halved and
stoned
½ tsp vanilla essence

100g/3½oz pistachios, chopped
120ml/½ cup water

Method:

Add all the ingredients, except the pistachios, into the slow cooker. Cover and leave to cook on low for 2-3 hours or until the apricots are soft and the liquid syrupy. Sprinkle the pistachios over the top and serve with low fat crème fraiche.

If the apricots are not very ripe you might need to add a little more sugar.

Ginger Plums With Greek Yoghurt

Serves 4

Ingredients:

900g/2lb plums, halved and
stoned
1 tbsp freshly grated ginger

3 tbsp runny honey
500ml/2 cups fat free Greek
yoghurt

Method:

Place all the ingredients, except the yoghurt, in the slow cooker
and combine well. Cover and leave to cook on low for 4-6 hours.
Add a little water during cooking if needed. Divide the yoghurt
into bowls and serve with the plums piled on top.

*Feel free to use ground ginger if you don't have any
fresh to hand.*

THE
Skinny **SLOW COOKER VEGETARIAN**
RECIPE BOOK

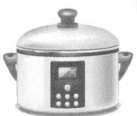

BREAKFASTS

Spanish Tortilla
Serves 4

325 CALORIES PER SERVING

Ingredients:

A dozen eggs, gently fork-whisked
One large onion, chopped
150g/5oz potatoes, peeled and cut into thin slices

Low cal cooking spray
Salt & pepper to taste.

Method:

Gently fry the onions and sliced potatoes in a little low cal spray for 5-10 mins. Spray the slow cooker with a little more oil and add all the ingredients. Combine well, season, cover and leave to cook on low for 4-6 hours.

This Spanish omelette makes a fantastic hearty start to the morning. It is also great served cold and cut into slices with a fresh green salad.

Multi Grain Breakfast

Serves 4

Ingredients:

25g/1oz rolled oats
75g/3oz bulgur wheat
100g/3 ½ oz brown rice
25g/1oz pearl barley
50g/2oz quinoa
150g/5oz chopped apple (no need to peel)

75g/3oz raisins
1 tsp ground cinnamon
1 tbsp vanilla extract
1lt/4 cups water
Sprinkle of nutmeg

Method:

Combine all the ingredients (except the nutmeg) well in the slow cooker and leave to cook on low for 6 to 8 hours with the lid tightly shut. Add more water if needed and stir well. Sprinkle with nutmeg after cooking.

Serve with soymilk and a drop of organic maple syrup to your taste.

This is a lovely way to start your day. The combination of grains in this dish make for a balanced multigrain start.

Fruit Granola
Serves 4

285
CALORIES
PER SERVING

Ingredients:

2 cups plain granola cereal
50g/2oz oatmeal
½ tsp cinnamon
½ tsp nutmeg (if you've got it)
1 tbsp brown sugar

1 tbsp runny honey
5 apples, sliced
50g/2oz sultanas
2 tsp low fat 'butter' spread
60ml/ ¼ cup water

Method:

Add all the ingredients to the slow cooker and combine well.
Leave to cook on low for 4-6 hours. Make sure the granola doesn't
burn, add a little more water if needed. Serve with milk if you like.

*This recipe is basically your favourite granola cereal
combined with fresh fruit and spices to fill your
kitchen with a lovely warming, welcoming aroma
in the morning. (Also lovely as a dessert with a little
more sugar and a dob of fresh cream).*

Morning Risotto
Serves 4

271
CALORIES
PER SERVING

Ingredients:

175g/6oz risotto rice
4 apples, sliced
150g/5oz sultanas
½ tsp cinnamon
½ tsp nutmeg
¼ tsp ground cloves

500ml/2 cups water
500ml/2 cups semi skimmed milk
1 tbsp brown sugar
1 tsp low fat 'butter' spread

Method:

Melt the butter in the slow cooker and add the rice. Stir to make sure it's all nicely coated then add all the other ingredients to the slow cooker. Cover and leave to cook on low for 4-6 hours or until the rice is tender. Add a little more milk during cooking if needed.

Another lovely breakfast alternative, which uses Italian rice to give the dish its base.

Vanilla Prunes
Serves 4

Ingredients:

750ml/3 cups water
350g/12oz pitted prunes
75g/3oz caster/fine sugar

2 tsp vanilla extract
1 tea bag

Method:

Boil the water and place in the warmed slow cooker with the teabag. After 3 minutes remove the teabag and discard. Add all the other ingredients to the pan, cover and leave to cook on low for 7-9 hours or until the prunes are tender and the liquid syrupy. Delicious served warm with fat free Greek yoghurt.

You should be left with tender prunes and syrup sauce which is delicious served with Greek yoghurt.

Banana Porridge Oats
Serves 4

Ingredients:

750ml/3 cups water
250ml/1 cup semi skimmed milk
3 tbsp brown sugar

½ tsp ground cinnamon
150g/5oz rolled porridge oats
3 bananas, sliced

Method:

Add the water, milk, oats, cinnamon and half the sugar to the slow cooker. Combine well, cover and leave to cook for 1-2 hours on low. You can leave it a little longer to thicken if needed, alternatively if it's a bit stodgy loosen up with some more milk. When the porridge is ready divide into bowls, add the sliced bananas and sprinkle with the remaining sugar.

Oats give you a hearty start and slowly release energy throughout the day.

A Real Cooked Breakfast

Serves 4

Ingredients:

4 vegetarian sausages
4 vine ripened tomatoes, halved
450g/1lb potatoes, peeled and cubed
4 portabella mushrooms, thickly sliced

60ml/¼ cup vegetable stock/broth
2 tsp wholegrain mustard
1 tbsp tomato puree/paste
1 onion, sliced
Low cal cooking oil
Salt & pepper to taste

Method:

Spray the slow cooker with a little low cal oil. Add all the ingredients, combine well, season, cover and leave to cook on low for 4-6 hours or until everything is cooked through and tender. Add a little more stock during cooking if needed.

This is a great healthier alternative to a fried full English breakfast.

Conversion Chart

Weights for dry ingredients:

Metric	Imperial
7g	¼ oz
15g	½ oz
20g	¾ oz
25g	1 oz
40g	1½oz
50g	2oz
60g	2½oz
75g	3oz
100g	3½oz
125g	4oz
140g	4½oz
150g	5oz
165g	5½oz
175g	6oz
200g	7oz
225g	8oz
250g	9oz
275g	10oz
300g	11oz
350g	12oz
375g	13oz
400g	14oz
425g	15oz
450g	1lb
500g	1lb 2oz
550g	1¼lb
600g	1lb 5oz
650g	1lb 7oz
675g	1½lb
700g	1lb 9oz
750g	1lb 11oz
800g	1¾lb
900g	2lb
1kg	2¼lb
1.1kg	2½lb
1.25kg	2¾lb
1.35kg	3lb
1.5kg	3lb 6oz
1.8kg	4lb
2kg	4½lb
2.25kg	5lb
2.5kg	5½lb
2.75kg	6lb

Conversion Chart
Liquid measures:

Metric	Imperial	Aus	US
25ml	1fl oz		
60ml	2fl oz	¼ cup	¼ cup
75ml	3fl oz		
100ml	3½fl oz		
120ml	4fl oz	½ cup	½ cup
150ml	5fl oz		
175ml	6fl oz	¾ cup	¾ cup
200ml	7fl oz		
250ml	8fl oz	1 cup	1 cup
300ml	10fl oz/½ pt	1¼ cups	
360ml	12fl oz		
400ml	14fl oz		
450ml	15fl oz	2 cups	2 cups/1 pint
600ml	1 pint	1 pint	2½ cups
750ml	1¼ pint		
900ml	1½ pints		
1 litre	1½ pints	1¾ pints	1 quart

Other CookNation Titles

You may also be interested in other titles in the CookNation series

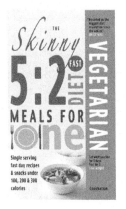

The Skinny 5:2 Fast Diet Vegetarian Meals For One
Single Serving Fast Day Recipes & Snacks Under 100, 200 & 300 Calories.

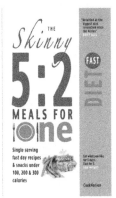

The Skinny 5:2 Fast Diet Meals For One
Single Serving Fast Day Recipes & Snacks Under 100, 200 & 300 Calories.

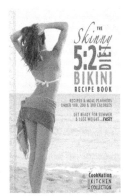

The Skinny 5:2 Bikini Diet Recipe Book
Recipes & Meal Planners Under 100, 200 & 300 Calories. Get Ready For Summer & Lose Weight... FAST!

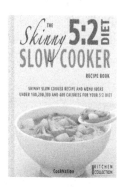

The Skinny 5:2 Slow Cooker Recipe Book
Skinny Slow Cooker Recipe And Menu Ideas Under 100, 200, 300 & 400 Calories For Your 5:2 Diet.

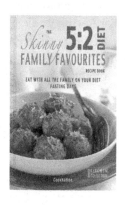

The Skinny 5:2 Family Favourites Recipe Book
(UK Edition)
Eat With All the Family On Your Diet Fasting Days

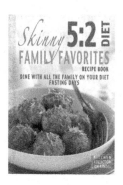

The Skinny 5:2 Family Favorites Recipe Book
(USA Edition)
Dine With All The Family On Your Diet Fasting Days

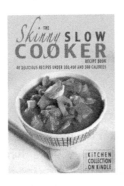

**The Skinny Slow Cooker
Recipe Book**
40 Delicious Recipes Under
300, 400 And 500 Calories.

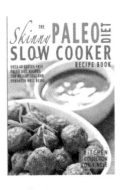

**The Skinny Paleo Diet Slow
Cooker Recipe Book**
Over 40 Gluten Free Paleo
Diet Recipes For Weight Loss
And Enhanced Well Being.

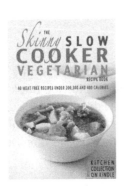

**The Skinny Slow Cooker
Vegetarian Recipe Book**
40 Delicious Recipes Under
200, 300 And 400 Calories.

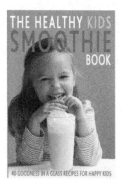

**The Healthy Kids
Smoothie Book**
40 Delicious Goodness
In A Glass Recipes for
Happy Kids.

Find all these great titles by searching under
'**CookNation**' on Amazon.

Review

If you enjoyed The Skinny Slow Cooker Vegetarian
Recipe Book we'd really appreciate your feedback.
Reviews help others decide if this is the right book for
them so a moment of your time would be appreciated.
Thank you.